RENAL DIET COOKBOOK
FOR SENIORS

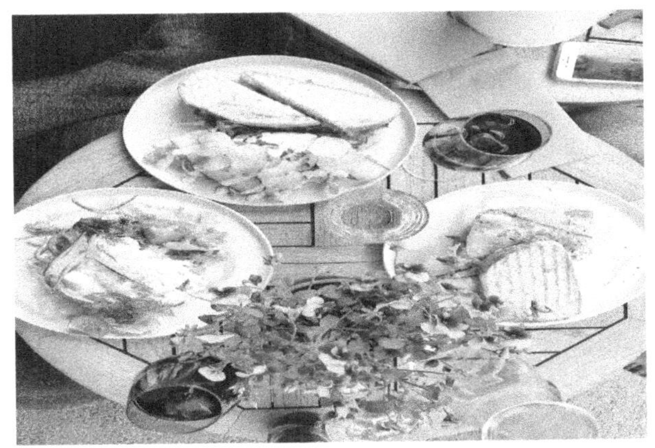

STEP-BY- STEP NUTRITIONAL GUIDE TO KIDNEY WELLNESS

JULIAN MORGAN

TABLE OF CONTENTS

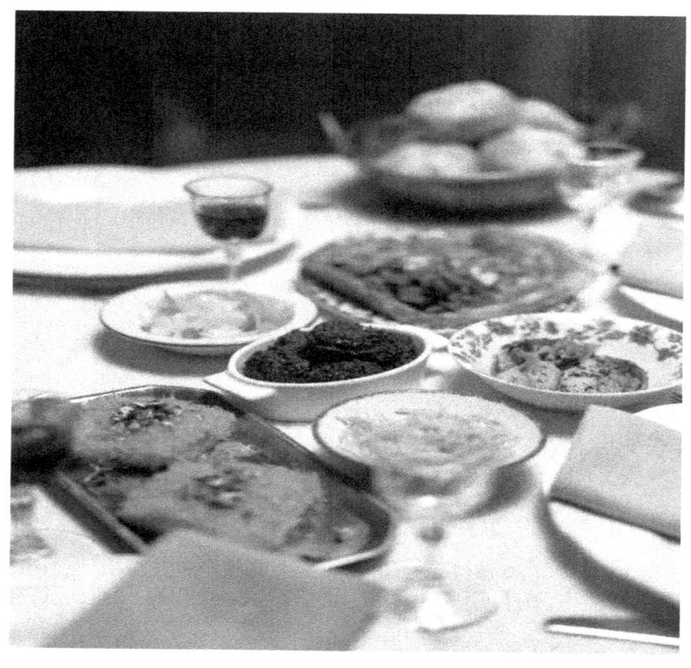

INTRODUCTION

Embark on a culinary journey tailored to elevate the health and vitality of our cherished seniors with the "Quick, Delicious, Nutritious - A Seniors' Renal Harmony Cookbook for Vibrant Health." In these pages, discover a symphony of flavors meticulously crafted to support renal well-being without compromising on the joy of savoring each meal. This culinary masterpiece is more than a collection of recipes; it's a guide to redefining how we nourish our bodies, proving that wholesome can be delectable. Prepare to be captivated by the fusion of culinary artistry and nutritional science, as we unlock the secrets to a renewed and invigorated life through the simple act of enjoying a delicious, health-conscious meal. Welcome to a world where every bite is a step towards well-being, where quick, delicious, and nutritious converge in a culinary celebration designed exclusively for our beloved seniors. Get ready to embark on a transformative gastronomic experience that transcends the ordinary, embracing a life of vitality, one delightful dish at a time.

Within these pages, you'll find more than just recipes; you'll uncover a roadmap to wellness, thoughtfully curated for the unique needs of seniors. Each dish is a testament to the belief that healthful eating need not sacrifice the pleasures of the palate. From the first sizzle in the pan to the last satisfying bite, this cookbook is a testament to the idea that nourishing the body can be a delightful and soul-enriching experience.

Prepare to be amazed as we redefine the possibilities of a renal diet, transforming it into a feast of culinary ingenuity. The recipes within are not just meals; they are a celebration of life, flavor, and the joy that comes from embracing a wholesome lifestyle.

As you turn these pages, imagine the delight of discovering quick, delicious, and nutritious creations that not only tantalize taste buds but also contribute to the overall well-being of our treasured seniors. It's a culinary odyssey where every recipe is a brushstroke on the canvas of health, and the resulting masterpiece is a life filled with energy, vitality, and the sheer pleasure of savoring exceptional meals.

So, fasten your apron, sharpen your knives, and get ready to embark on a culinary adventure that transcends the ordinary—because good health should never mean compromising on the joy of a truly satisfying meal. Welcome to a world where the kitchen becomes a haven of well-being, and every recipe is a step towards a more vibrant, flavorful life.

CHAPTER ONE

WELCOMING SENIORS TO RENAL HEALTH AND CULINARY WELLNESS

As we embark on a journey to embrace renal health and culinary wellness for seniors, it's crucial to recognize the significance of nurturing our bodies as we age. This chapter serves as a warm introduction, inviting seniors into the realm of wholesome living tailored to support kidney function and overall well-being.

Embracing Renal Wellness

Understanding the Importance:
Aging gracefully involves caring for every aspect of our health, and the kidneys play a pivotal role in this journey. Seniors, more than ever, need to be conscious of their renal health to maintain vitality and a high quality of life. This chapter unfolds the layers of understanding renal wellness, providing insights into the functions of the kidneys and their impact on our overall health.

Navigating Culinary Wellness:

The kitchen becomes a haven for seniors seeking to prioritize their renal health. It's not just about what we eat; it's about the art of crafting meals that are both delicious and beneficial. We explore the concept of culinary wellness, where every ingredient is chosen with care to contribute to optimal renal function.

The Journey Begins: Senior-Specific Nutritional Needs

Tailoring Diets to Seniors:
Seniors have unique nutritional needs, and addressing these needs is key to promoting their well-being. We delve into the specifics of senior nutrition, understanding the nutrients that become even more crucial as we age. From protein requirements to fluid intake, we guide seniors on tailoring their diets to ensure they get the nutrition essential for renal health.

Crafting a Renal-Friendly Pantry: Navigating Renal-Friendly Ingredients

A Pantry Makeover:
Transforming the kitchen starts with the right ingredients. This section offers a comprehensive guide to navigating the aisles with renal health in mind. From whole grains to kidney-friendly proteins, seniors will discover a wealth of options to elevate

their culinary creations while supporting their kidneys.

The Power of Fresh Produce:
Fruits and vegetables become the stars of the show in a renal-friendly kitchen. We explore the vibrant world of produce, highlighting choices that bring flavor and nutrition to the forefront. Seniors will learn how to incorporate these ingredients into their meals, fostering a love for fresh, wholesome eating.

Energizing Mornings: Breakfasts to Kickstart the Day

Start the Day Right:
Breakfast isn't just a meal; it's a rejuvenating experience. We present a collection of renal-friendly breakfast ideas that burst with flavor and nourishment. From hearty oatmeal to protein-packed omelets, seniors will find inspiration to kickstart their day with energy and vitality.

Midday Nourishment: Wholesome Lunches for Optimal Wellness

Balancing Act:
Lunch becomes a delightful balancing act of flavors, textures, and nutrients. We explore lunch options that cater to renal health without compromising on taste. Seniors will discover

satisfying meals that keep them fueled throughout the day, promoting optimal wellness.

Evening Indulgences: Flavorful Dinners with Renal Health in Mind

Culinary Delights at Dinnertime:
Dinner is a time for culinary exploration, and this section introduces seniors to a repertoire of renal-friendly dinner options. From succulent fish dishes to hearty vegetarian stews, we showcase meals that are not only good for the kidneys but also a celebration of diverse flavors.

Tempting Bites: Snacks and Sides for Satisfying Cravings

Craving Satisfaction Without Compromise:
Snacking takes center stage as we explore renal-friendly options that satisfy cravings while contributing to kidney health. Seniors will discover a variety of snacks and sides that make mindful eating a pleasure.

Sweet Treats: Desserts Without Compromising Health

Indulgence with Care:

Desserts need not be off-limits. In this section, we present sweet indulgences crafted with kidney health in mind. From fruit-based delights to inventive low-sugar treats, seniors can savor the joy of desserts without compromising their well-being.

Hydration and Kidney Support: Beverages for a Healthy Balance

Quenching Thirst, Supporting Kidneys:
Proper hydration is vital for renal health. We explore beverages that go beyond just quenching thirst, offering support to the kidneys. Seniors will discover refreshing options that contribute to their overall well-being.

Practical Tips and Tricks: Meal Planning for Renal Health

Efficiency in the Kitchen:
Meal planning becomes a breeze with practical tips and tricks designed for seniors. From efficient grocery shopping to batch cooking, we guide seniors on simplifying their culinary routines while prioritizing renal health.

Navigating Dining Out: A Guide for Seniors

Eating Out Without Compromise:
Seniors need not feel restricted when dining out.
This section provides a guide on navigating
restaurant menus while making choices that align
with renal health goals. From smart menu
selections to communication tips, seniors can enjoy
dining out with confidence.

Beyond the Plate: Lifestyle Habits for Improved Renal Function

Holistic Approaches to Health:
Renal health extends beyond the plate, and we
explore lifestyle habits that contribute to improved
kidney function. From staying active to managing
stress, seniors will find holistic approaches to
enhance their overall well-being.

Recipes at a Glance: Quick Reference Guide

Effortless Access to Culinary Delights:
This chapter concludes with a quick reference
guide, offering seniors easy access to their favorite
renal-friendly recipes. A handy resource for busy
days or moments of culinary inspiration.

Finding What You Need: Index for Easy Recipe Retrieval

Efficiency in Exploration:

To make this renal diet cookbook truly user-friendly, we provide a detailed index for easy recipe retrieval. Seniors can quickly locate their desired recipes, ensuring a seamless and enjoyable cooking experience.
As we embark on this journey of renal health and culinary wellness for seniors, let the kitchen become a place of nourishment, creativity, and joy—a space where every meal is a celebration of life and vitality.

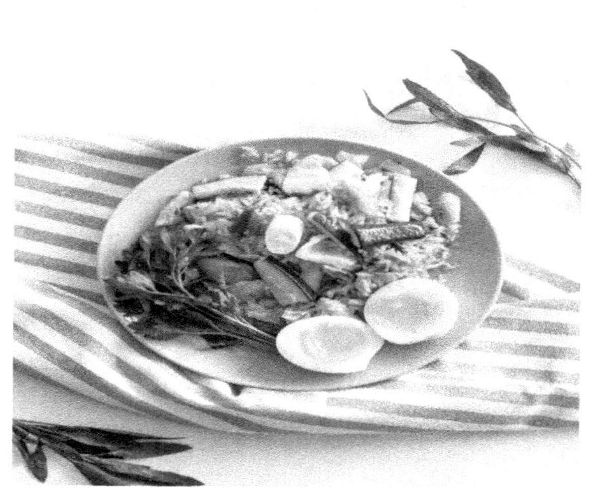

CHAPTER TWO

UNDERSTANDING RENAL HEALTH

- Exploring the Essentials of Kidney Function

The kidneys play a crucial role in maintaining the body's overall health by filtering and eliminating waste products and excess fluids. As individuals age, the efficiency of kidney function may diminish, making it imperative to adopt a renal-friendly diet. A renal diet cookbook for seniors becomes an essential resource in managing kidney health through nutrition.

Understanding Kidney Function:
The kidneys are responsible for filtering blood, removing waste products, and regulating fluid balance. They play a vital role in maintaining electrolyte levels, controlling blood pressure, and

producing hormones that influence red blood cell production. As people age, the kidneys may experience a decline in function, leading to conditions such as chronic kidney disease (CKD).

Challenges of Aging Kidneys:
Seniors often face challenges related to kidney health, such as decreased blood flow to the kidneys, reduced number of functional nephrons (the filtering units of the kidneys), and changes in hormone levels affecting fluid and electrolyte balance. These factors contribute to a higher susceptibility to kidney-related issues, making dietary adjustments crucial for overall well-being.

Renal Diet Basics:
A renal diet, also known as a kidney-friendly diet, focuses on managing the intake of certain nutrients to alleviate stress on the kidneys. Key components of a renal diet include controlling sodium, phosphorus, potassium, and fluid intake. These dietary modifications aim to ease the kidneys' workload and

minimize the risk of complications associated with impaired kidney function.

Sodium Restriction:
Reducing sodium intake is a cornerstone of a renal diet. Excessive sodium can lead to fluid retention and increased blood pressure, putting additional strain on the kidneys. A renal diet cookbook for seniors emphasizes the use of herbs, spices, and other flavorings to enhance taste without relying on high-sodium ingredients.

Phosphorus Management:
High levels of phosphorus in the blood can contribute to bone and cardiovascular issues in individuals with kidney problems. Renal-friendly recipes for seniors often include guidelines on choosing foods lower in phosphorus, such as lean proteins, grains, and vegetables. Additionally, the cookbook may provide creative ways to limit the use of high-phosphorus additives in cooking.

Potassium Control:

Seniors with kidney concerns need to monitor potassium intake, as imbalances can affect heart function. A renal diet cookbook offers recipes incorporating fruits and vegetables with lower potassium content, while still ensuring a nutritionally balanced diet. Cooking techniques that leach potassium from certain foods, such as boiling, may also be highlighted.

Fluid Regulation:

Controlling the amount of liquids consumed is essential for those whose renal function is impaired. A renal diet cookbook may provide recipes that account for both liquid and solid components, helping seniors maintain a balance that aligns with their prescribed fluid restrictions. This includes incorporating hydrating foods while being mindful of high-fluid ingredients.

Balancing Nutrient Intake:

Apart from specific nutrient restrictions, a renal diet cookbook for seniors emphasizes the importance of maintaining adequate nutrition. This involves incorporating a variety of nutrient-dense foods, ensuring sufficient protein intake from high-quality sources, and managing portion sizes to meet individual dietary needs.

Adapting Traditional Recipes:
One of the strengths of a renal diet cookbook lies in its ability to adapt traditional recipes to meet kidney-friendly requirements. This allows seniors to enjoy familiar flavors and meals while adhering to dietary restrictions. The cookbook may offer tips on ingredient substitutions, cooking methods, and portion control to align with renal health guidelines.

Educational Component:
Beyond providing recipes, a renal diet cookbook serves as an educational tool. It empowers seniors with information about the nutritional content of different foods and encourages informed

decision-making. Understanding the impact of dietary choices on kidney health enables seniors to actively participate in managing their well-being.

In conclusion, a renal diet cookbook for seniors is a valuable resource in navigating the complexities of kidney health through nutrition. By focusing on sodium, phosphorus, potassium, fluid intake, and overall nutrient balance, these cookbooks contribute to the well-being of seniors with compromised kidney function. The combination of practical recipes and educational content empowers individuals to make informed choices, promoting a healthier lifestyle tailored to their specific needs.

CHAPTER THREE

<u>SENIOR-SPECIFIC NUTRITIONAL NEEDS</u>

- Tailoring Dietary Choices for Aging Well

As individuals age, dietary choices become increasingly significant in maintaining overall health and well-being. For seniors, especially those with compromised kidney function, a tailored approach to nutrition is essential. A renal diet cookbook for seniors emerges as a valuable tool, offering insights and recipes that cater to the specific needs of aging individuals, promoting kidney health and overall vitality.

The Aging Process and Nutrition:

Aging is accompanied by various physiological changes that influence nutrient absorption, metabolism, and overall nutritional requirements. Reduced muscle mass, changes in digestion, and altered taste and smell perception can impact dietary habits. A renal diet cookbook takes into account these age-related changes, providing recipes that are not only kidney-friendly but also address the unique nutritional needs of seniors.

Balancing Protein Intake:

Protein is crucial for maintaining muscle mass and supporting overall health, yet seniors may face challenges in protein utilization. A renal diet cookbook for seniors addresses this by including recipes that incorporate high-quality protein sources while managing phosphorus levels. It guides seniors in choosing lean meats, dairy alternatives, and plant-based proteins to meet their protein requirements without putting excess strain on the kidneys.

Calcium and Vitamin D Considerations:

Maintaining bone health becomes increasingly important as individuals age. A renal diet cookbook recognizes the need for adequate calcium and vitamin D intake while considering phosphorus restrictions. It offers recipes featuring foods rich in these nutrients, such as low-phosphorus dairy alternatives, fortified cereals, and green leafy vegetables. This ensures that seniors can enjoy flavorful meals that contribute to their bone health without compromising kidney function.

Micronutrient-Rich Options:

Aging individuals often require a higher intake of certain vitamins and minerals to support immune function and cognitive health. A renal diet cookbook for seniors includes recipes rich in antioxidants, vitamins, and minerals to meet these specific needs. Incorporating a variety of colorful fruits and vegetables, nuts, and whole grains, these recipes contribute to overall well-being and help seniors age gracefully.

Fiber for Digestive Health:

Digestive issues can become more prevalent as individuals age. Including fiber-rich foods in the diet becomes crucial for maintaining digestive health. A renal diet cookbook introduces recipes that incorporate high-fiber ingredients such as fruits, vegetables, and whole grains. These recipes not only support digestion but also contribute to heart health and weight management, addressing common concerns for seniors.

Sodium Consciousness:

Managing sodium intake becomes increasingly important with age, especially for those with compromised kidney function. A renal diet cookbook for seniors emphasizes the importance of reducing sodium while enhancing flavor through herbs and spices. By providing flavorful recipes that prioritize low-sodium ingredients, the cookbook helps seniors maintain a heart-healthy diet while safeguarding their kidney health.

Hydration Strategies:

Dehydration is a common concern for seniors, and maintaining adequate fluid intake is essential. A renal diet cookbook offers recipes that incorporate hydrating foods and suggests ways to meet fluid needs without overburdening the kidneys. This includes recipes for soups, stews, and fruit-infused beverages that contribute to overall hydration while aligning with renal health guidelines.

Personalized Dietary Approaches:

Every senior is unique, and a one-size-fits-all approach to nutrition may not be suitable. A renal diet cookbook recognizes the importance of individualized dietary choices and provides guidance on adapting recipes to meet specific needs. This may include adjusting portion sizes, making ingredient substitutions based on personal preferences or dietary restrictions, and encouraging a flexible approach to ensure that seniors can enjoy meals that suit their tastes and health requirements.

Culinary Creativity and Social Connection:

Beyond nutrition, a renal diet cookbook for seniors encourages culinary creativity and social connection. Cooking and sharing meals with others can be a source of joy and fulfillment. The cookbook provides ideas for adapting recipes for social gatherings, allowing seniors to maintain a connection with friends and family while adhering to their dietary restrictions.

In summary, In the journey of aging well, nutrition plays a pivotal role, and a renal diet cookbook for seniors serves as a valuable resource in this endeavor. By addressing the specific nutritional needs of aging individuals, balancing protein intake, considering bone health, emphasizing micronutrient-rich options, promoting digestive health, and addressing hydration concerns, these cookbooks contribute to a holistic approach to senior nutrition. With a focus on personalized dietary choices, culinary creativity, and social connection, a renal diet cookbook empowers seniors to make informed decisions about their diet, supporting their overall well-being and enhancing their quality of life.

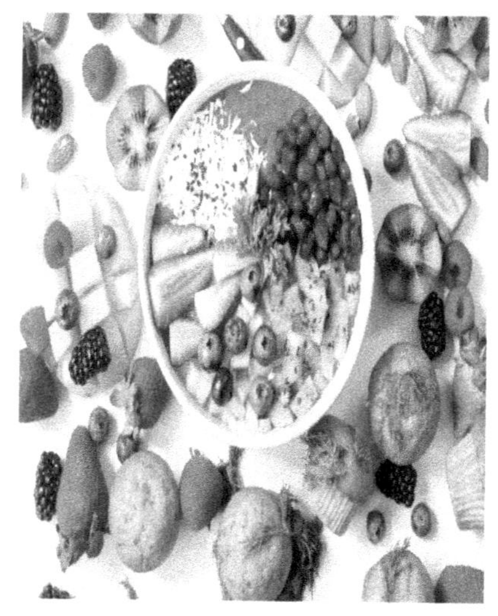

CHAPTER FOUR

NAVIGATING RENAL-FRIENDLY INGREDIENTS

- A Comprehensive Guide to Wholesome Choices

Navigating renal-friendly ingredients is a crucial aspect of creating a wholesome and nutritious diet for seniors with compromised kidney function. A renal diet cookbook tailored for seniors provides a comprehensive guide to making wholesome choices while considering the specific needs of aging individuals. This guide delves into key considerations when selecting ingredients, offering insights into the nutritional value of various foods and their impact on kidney health.

Understanding Renal-Friendly Ingredients:

A renal-friendly diet focuses on managing sodium, phosphorus, potassium, and fluid intake to alleviate stress on the kidneys. A renal diet cookbook for seniors serves as a roadmap for incorporating ingredients that align with these dietary restrictions while ensuring a balanced and flavorful culinary experience.

Low-Sodium Alternatives:

Reducing sodium intake is a cornerstone of a renal diet. A comprehensive renal diet cookbook guides seniors toward low-sodium alternatives. This includes using fresh herbs, spices, and salt-free seasonings to enhance flavor without compromising kidney health. It also educates seniors on selecting low-sodium versions of condiments and processed foods, promoting a heart-healthy and kidney-friendly approach to seasoning.

Lean Protein Sources:

Protein is essential for maintaining muscle mass and overall health, but seniors with kidney concerns need to be mindful of phosphorus levels. The cookbook highlights lean protein sources such as skinless poultry, fish, and plant-based proteins like tofu and legumes. It provides creative recipes that incorporate these proteins in delicious and kidney-friendly ways, ensuring seniors meet their nutritional needs without overburdening their kidneys.

Phosphorus Management:

A comprehensive guide within the renal diet cookbook educates seniors on managing phosphorus intake. This involves choosing grains, bread, and cereals with lower phosphorus content and minimizing the consumption of high-phosphorus additives. By understanding the phosphorus content of various foods, seniors can make informed choices to support their kidney health while still enjoying a diverse and satisfying diet.

Potassium-Controlled Options:

Seniors need to manage potassium intake to prevent complications such as irregular heartbeats. The renal diet cookbook provides insights into selecting fruits and vegetables with lower potassium content, such as apples, berries, and cauliflower. It also offers cooking techniques that help leach potassium from certain foods, allowing seniors to enjoy a variety of flavorful options while adhering to their dietary restrictions.

Hydrating Foods:

Maintaining adequate fluid intake is essential, and a renal diet cookbook emphasizes incorporating hydrating foods. This includes recipes with high-water-content ingredients like cucumbers, watermelon, and soups made with low-sodium broth. The cookbook provides a variety of options to help seniors meet their fluid needs while considering the impact on kidney function.

Whole Grains and Fiber-Rich Choices:

A wholesome renal diet encourages the consumption of whole grains and fiber-rich foods for digestive health. The cookbook introduces seniors to a variety of whole grains such as quinoa, brown rice, and whole wheat pasta. It also includes recipes with fiber-rich ingredients like fruits, vegetables, and legumes, promoting overall well-being and supporting digestive function.

Educational Insights into Ingredient Selection:

Beyond providing recipes, a comprehensive renal diet cookbook serves as an educational resource. It offers insights into the nutritional content of different ingredients, enabling seniors to make informed decisions about their food choices. By understanding how specific ingredients affect kidney health, seniors can confidently adapt recipes to suit their preferences and dietary needs.

Portion Control and Nutrient Balance:

Seniors often face challenges related to portion control and maintaining a nutrient balance. The cookbook addresses these concerns by providing guidelines on portion sizes and ensuring recipes offer a well-balanced nutritional profile. This empowers seniors to enjoy satisfying meals without exceeding their dietary restrictions, promoting overall health and well-being.

Adapting Familiar Flavors:

A key aspect of the renal diet cookbook is its ability to adapt familiar flavors to meet kidney-friendly requirements. It introduces seniors to ingredient substitutions and cooking methods that maintain the essence of their favorite dishes while aligning with dietary restrictions. This adaptability ensures that seniors can enjoy a diverse and satisfying culinary experience, enhancing their overall quality of life.

Conclusion:

In conclusion, a comprehensive guide to renal-friendly ingredients within a renal diet cookbook for seniors is an invaluable resource for navigating the complexities of dietary choices. By emphasizing low-sodium alternatives, lean protein sources, phosphorus management, potassium-controlled options, hydrating foods, whole grains, and fiber-rich choices, the cookbook empowers seniors to make wholesome and informed decisions about their nutrition. With educational insights, guidance on portion control, and the ability to adapt familiar flavors, the cookbook becomes a practical tool for seniors to embrace a kidney-friendly lifestyle that promotes their overall health and well-being.

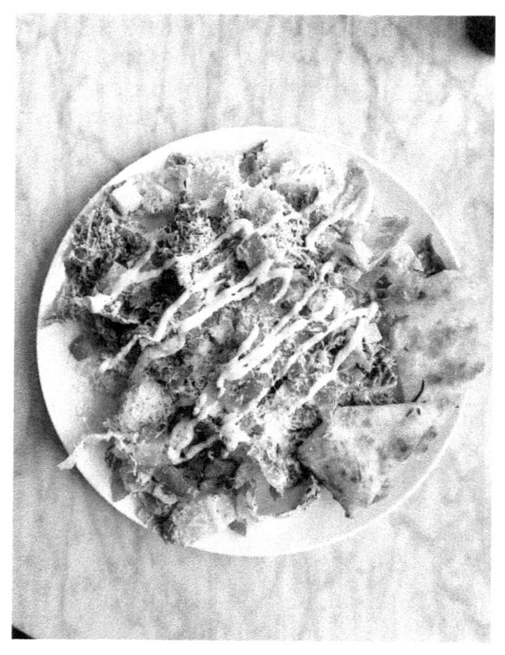

CHAPTER FIVE

BREAKFAST TO ENERGIZE YOUR DAY

- Morning Delights Packed with Nutritional Power

Embracing the day with morning delights not only kickstarts energy levels but also sets the tone for a wholesome and nutritious day. For seniors following a renal diet, a specialized cookbook offers morning recipes that are not only delicious but also packed with nutritional power to support kidney health. Let's explore five delightful recipes along with instructions, designed to nourish seniors on their wellness journey.

1. Berry Bliss Breakfast Parfait:

Ingredients:

1/2 cup fresh blueberries

1/2 cup sliced strawberries

1/2 cup low-fat Greek yogurt

1/4 cup chopped walnuts (unsalted)

1 teaspoon honey (optional)

Instructions:

Half of the Greek yogurt should be layered in a glass or dish.
Add a portion of blueberries and strawberries on top

of the yogurt.

Sprinkle a portion of chopped walnuts over the

berries.

With the remaining ingredients, repeat the stacking procedure.
If desired, drizzle some honey over the top for further sweetness.

Serve chilled and enjoy a refreshing and protein-packed breakfast.

2. Quinoa and Fruit Breakfast Bowl:
Ingredients:

1/2 cup cooked quinoa
1/4 cup diced mango
1/4 cup diced pineapple
1/4 cup sliced kiwi
1 tablespoon chopped mint leaves
1 tablespoon unsweetened coconut flakes
Instructions:

In a bowl, combine cooked quinoa and diced fruits.
Sprinkle chopped mint leaves and coconut flakes over the mixture.
Gently toss the ingredients to evenly distribute flavors.
Serve at room temperature and savor the delightful combination of textures and tropical flavors.

3. Spinach and Feta Omelette:

Ingredients:

2 large eggs

1/4 cup fresh spinach, chopped

2 tablespoons crumbled feta cheese

1 tablespoon olive oil

Salt and pepper to taste

Instructions:

In a bowl, whisk the eggs and season with salt and pepper.

Heat olive oil in a non-stick skillet over medium heat.

Add chopped spinach to the skillet and sauté until wilted.

Pour the whisked eggs over the spinach, allowing them to set slightly.

Sprinkle crumbled feta cheese over one half of the omelette.

The remaining half should be folded over the filling to form a semicircle.

Cook until the eggs are fully set.

Slide the omelette onto a plate, and serve a

nutrient-rich breakfast that's high in protein and flavor.

4. Apple Cinnamon Chia Pudding:

Ingredients:

2 tablespoons chia seeds

1/2 cup unsweetened almond milk

1/2 teaspoon ground cinnamon

1/2 apple, diced

1 tablespoon chopped almonds (unsalted)

Instructions:

In a bowl, mix chia seeds and almond milk.

Allow it to sit for ten minutes, giving it periodic stirs.

Stir in ground cinnamon to the chia mixture.

Layer the chia pudding with diced apples in a serving glass.

Repeat the layers, finishing with a sprinkle of chopped almonds on top.

Refrigerate for at least two hours or overnight for a delicious and fiber-packed breakfast.

5. Whole Grain Pancakes with Berries:

Ingredients:

1/2 cup whole wheat flour

1/2 teaspoon baking powder

1/4 teaspoon cinnamon

1/2 cup low-fat buttermilk

1 egg

1 tablespoon melted unsalted butter

Half a cup of mixed berries, such as strawberries, raspberries, or blueberries

Instructions:

In a bowl, whisk together whole wheat flour, baking powder, and cinnamon.

Combine melted butter, egg, and buttermilk in a separate basin.
Stir the dry and wet components together until they are well blended.
Over medium heat, preheat a nonstick skillet or griddle.
Pour 1/4 cup of batter onto the griddle for each pancake.

Fry until surface bubbles appear, then turn and finish cooking the other side.

Serve the pancakes with a generous topping of mixed berries for a delightful, whole-grain breakfast option.

6. Avocado and Salmon Toast:

Ingredients:

1 slice whole-grain bread

1/4 ripe avocado, mashed

2 ounces smoked salmon

1 teaspoon capers

Fresh dill for garnish

Instructions:

Toast the whole-grain bread to your liking.

On the toast, equally distribute the mashed avocado.

Drape smoked salmon over the avocado.

Sprinkle capers on top for a burst of flavor.

Garnish with fresh dill.

This nutrient-packed toast provides healthy fats and

omega-3s, making it a satisfying and kidney-friendly

breakfast option.

7. Mediterranean Veggie Scramble:

Ingredients:

2 large eggs

1/4 cup cherry tomatoes, halved

2 tablespoons diced bell peppers (assorted colors)

2 tablespoons crumbled feta cheese

1 tablespoon chopped fresh basil

Olive oil for cooking

Instructions:

In a pan, warm up a tiny bit of olive oil over medium

heat.

Saute diced bell peppers until slightly softened.

Whisk the eggs and pour them into the pan with the

peppers.

Add cherry tomatoes to the eggs.

Stir gently until the eggs are almost set, then add crumbled feta and chopped basil.

Cook the eggs until they are well set.

Serve this Mediterranean-inspired scramble for a protein-rich and flavorful breakfast.

8. Oatmeal with Mixed Berries and Almonds:

Ingredients:

1/2 cup old-fashioned oats

1 cup water or low-fat milk

1/2 cup mixed berries (strawberries, blueberries, raspberries)

1 tablespoon chopped almonds (unsalted)

1 teaspoon honey (optional)

Instructions:

Cook the oats with water or milk according to package instructions.

Once cooked, top with mixed berries and chopped almonds.

Drizzle with honey for added sweetness if desired.

Stir the ingredients together and enjoy a warm and comforting bowl of oatmeal rich in fiber, antioxidants, and essential nutrients.

9. Sweet Potato and Spinach Hash:

Ingredients:

1 medium sweet potato, peeled and grated

1 cup fresh spinach, chopped

1/4 cup diced red onion

1 tablespoon olive oil

2 eggs (optional)

Salt and pepper to taste

Instructions:

1. In a pan over medium heat, warm the olive oil.

2. Add the diced red onion and shredded sweet potato, and sauté until the sweet potato is soft.

3. Stir in chopped spinach and cook until wilted.

4. If desired, create wells in the hash and crack eggs into them.

5. Cover the skillet and cook until the eggs are cooked to your liking.

6. Season with salt and pepper and serve this nutrient-packed hash as a hearty and flavorful breakfast.

10. Banana Nut Smoothie Bowl:

Ingredients:

- 1 ripe banana
- 1/2 cup low-fat Greek yogurt
- 1/4 cup chopped walnuts (unsalted)
- 1 tablespoon chia seeds
- Drizzle of honey for sweetness (optional)
- Fresh banana slices for garnish

Instructions:
1. In a blender, combine ripe banana and low-fat Greek yogurt.
2. Blend until smooth and creamy.
3. Pour the smoothie into a bowl.
4. Top with chopped walnuts, chia seeds, and fresh banana slices.
5. Drizzle with honey for added sweetness if desired.
6. Enjoy a satisfying and protein-rich smoothie bowl that's easy on the kidneys and bursting with flavor.

Conclusion:
Expanding the repertoire of renal-friendly morning delights, these additional recipes bring diversity to

the breakfast table while prioritizing kidney health. From a nutrient-packed Avocado and Salmon Toast to the comforting Sweet Potato and Spinach Hash, these recipes cater to seniors following a renal diet, providing a delicious start to their day. Incorporating a variety of flavors, textures, and essential nutrients, these breakfast options ensure that seniors can enjoy a wholesome and satisfying morning meal while supporting their overall well-being.

CHAPTER SIX

WHOLESOME LUNCHES FOR OPTIMAL WELLNESS

- Midday Nourishment with a Focus on Renal Health

Lunch is a crucial meal for seniors following a renal diet, as it plays a significant role in maintaining kidney health. A renal diet aims to manage the intake of certain nutrients, such as sodium, potassium, and phosphorus, to support kidney function. Here's a comprehensive guide to midday nourishment with a focus on renal health within a senior renal diet cookbook:

1. Protein Management:
    - Choose lean protein sources like skinless poultry, fish, and eggs to provide essential amino acids without overloading on phosphorus.

- Incorporate plant-based proteins like beans, lentils, and tofu to add variety while keeping protein intake in check.

2. Balanced Carbohydrates:

- Opt for whole grains like brown rice, quinoa, and whole wheat bread to ensure a steady release of energy without contributing excessive phosphorus.

- Control portion sizes of starchy vegetables to manage potassium levels.

3. Low Sodium Options:

- Reduce salt intake by using herbs, spices, and low-sodium seasonings to enhance flavor.

- Choose fresh, unprocessed foods over pre-packaged or canned options to minimize sodium content.

4. Fluid Intake:
   - Stay mindful of fluid intake, as seniors with kidney issues may need to monitor fluid retention.
   - Include hydrating foods like fruits and vegetables with high water content.

5. Phosphorus Awareness:
   - Limit high-phosphorus foods such as dairy products, nuts, and seeds.
   - Soak, leach, or choose lower phosphorus alternatives for certain foods to reduce phosphorus content.

6. Vegetable Variety:

   o   Emphasize a colorful array of
       vegetables to provide essential
       vitamins and minerals while
       managing potassium levels.

   o   Cook vegetables using methods
       that reduce potassium content,
       such as boiling.

7. Dessert Delights:

   o   Explore renal-friendly dessert
       options like fruit sorbets, gelatin,
       and angel food cake.

   o   Substitute high-phosphorus
       ingredients in traditional recipes
       to create kidney-friendly treats.

8. Beverage Choices:

   o   Encourage hydration with herbal
       teas, diluted fruit juices, and
       homemade flavored water.

- Limit caffeinated and high-sugar beverages to promote overall health.

9. Monitoring Portion Sizes:
   - Keep portion sizes moderate to avoid overloading the kidneys with excess nutrients.
   - Use smaller plates to create visually satisfying meals without exceeding dietary restrictions.

10. Consultation with Healthcare Professionals:
    - Regularly consult with healthcare professionals, including dietitians and doctors, to tailor the renal diet to individual needs.
    - Adjust the meal plan based on any changes in health status or medication.

Creating a midday meal within the framework of a renal diet for seniors requires thoughtful consideration of nutrient balance and portion control. By incorporating a variety of renal-friendly foods and staying vigilant about specific dietary restrictions, seniors can enjoy a delicious and nourishing lunch while supporting their renal health.

Below are few recipes

1. Grilled Lemon Herb Chicken:
    - Ingredients: Skinless chicken breast, lemon juice, garlic, rosemary, thyme.
    - Method: Marinate chicken in lemon juice, garlic, and herbs, then grill until fully cooked.
2. Quinoa Salad with Roasted Vegetables:
    - Ingredients: Quinoa, bell peppers, zucchini, cherry tomatoes, olive oil.
    - Method: Roast vegetables, mix with cooked quinoa, and drizzle with olive oil.
3. Salmon and Asparagus Parcels:
    - Ingredients: Salmon fillets, asparagus, lemon slices, dill.

- o Method: Wrap salmon and asparagus in foil with lemon slices and dill, bake until done.

4. Vegetarian Lentil Soup:
   - o Ingredients: Lentils, carrots, celery, onion, low-sodium vegetable broth.
   - o Method: Simmer lentils and vegetables in broth until tender for a hearty soup.

5. Spinach and Feta Stuffed Chicken:
   - o Ingredients: Chicken breast, spinach, feta cheese, garlic.
   - o Method: Stuff chicken with sautéed spinach and feta, then bake until golden.

6. Brown Rice Stir-Fry with Tofu and Veggies:

- ○ Ingredients: Brown rice, tofu, broccoli, bell peppers, low-sodium soy sauce.
- ○ Method: Stir-fry tofu and vegetables, toss with cooked brown rice and soy sauce.

7. Herb-Roasted Turkey Breast:
- ○ Ingredients: Turkey breast, olive oil, thyme, sage, garlic.
- ○ Method: Rub turkey with herbs and roast until the internal temperature is safe.

8. Egg Salad Lettuce Wraps:
- ○ Ingredients: Hard-boiled eggs, Greek yogurt, celery, lettuce leaves.

o   Method: Mix eggs, yogurt, and celery for a filling, low-phosphorus salad, then wrap in lettuce leaves.

9. Mushroom and Spinach Risotto:

o   Ingredients: Arborio rice, mushrooms, spinach, low-sodium vegetable broth.

o   Method: Sauté mushrooms and spinach, then cook rice slowly in vegetable broth for a creamy risotto.

10. Baked Cod with Lemon and Herbs:

o   Ingredients: Cod fillets, lemon juice, parsley, dill, garlic.

o   Method: Season cod with herbs and lemon juice, then bake until flaky and tender.

Remember to adapt portion sizes and ingredients based on individual dietary needs and consult with healthcare professionals for personalized advice. These recipes offer a variety of flavors and textures while adhering to the principles of a renal diet for senior health.

CHAPTER SEVEN

<u>FLAVORFUL DINNERS WITH RENAL HEALTH IN MIND</u>

- **Evening Meals that Prioritize Kidney Function.**

1. Baked Lemon Garlic Tilapia:

    o Ingredients: Tilapia fillets, lemon, garlic, olive oil.

    o Method: Marinate tilapia in lemon, garlic, and olive oil, then bake until flaky.

2. Vegetable and Chicken Kebabs:

    o Ingredients: Chicken breast, bell peppers, cherry tomatoes, onion.

    o Method: Skewer chicken and vegetables, grill until chicken is cooked through.

3. Cauliflower and Chickpea Curry:

- Ingredients: Cauliflower, chickpeas, tomatoes, curry spices.
- Method: Simmer cauliflower and chickpeas in a tomato-based curry sauce.

4. Turkey and Sweet Potato Casserole:
   - Ingredients: Ground turkey, sweet potatoes, onion, low-sodium broth.
   - Method: Brown turkey, layer with sliced sweet potatoes, and bake with broth until tender.

5. Shrimp and Broccoli Stir-Fry:
   - Ingredients: Shrimp, broccoli, snap peas, low-sodium soy sauce.

- o Method: Stir-fry shrimp and vegetables, add soy sauce for a flavorful dish.

6. Lemon Herb Quinoa with Grilled Veggies:
    - o Ingredients: Quinoa, zucchini, eggplant, lemon, herbs.
    - o Method: Grill vegetables, mix with cooked quinoa, and dress with lemon and herbs.

7. Slow Cooker Beef Stew:
    - o Ingredients: Lean beef, carrots, celery, potatoes, low-sodium beef broth.
    - o Method: Combine ingredients in a slow cooker for a hearty and kidney-friendly stew.

8. Eggplant and Tomato Bake:

- o Ingredients: Eggplant, tomatoes, garlic, basil.
- o Method: Layer sliced eggplant and tomatoes, bake with garlic and basil until tender.

9. Spaghetti Squash with Turkey Bolognese:

- o Ingredients: Spaghetti squash, ground turkey, tomato sauce.
- o Method: Roast spaghetti squash, top with turkey bolognese made with low-phosphorus tomato sauce.

10. Chicken and Vegetable Skillet:

- o Ingredients: Chicken thighs, green beans, mushrooms, low-sodium broth.

o Method: Sear chicken, add vegetables and broth, simmer until chicken is cooked.

11. Salmon Patties with Dill Sauce:

o Ingredients: Canned salmon, breadcrumbs, egg, dill, Greek yogurt.

o Method: Mix ingredients, form into patties, and pan-fry. Serve with dill sauce.

12. Mediterranean Chickpea Salad:

o Ingredients: Chickpeas, cucumber, cherry tomatoes, feta cheese, olive oil.

o Method: Toss ingredients together for a refreshing and kidney-friendly salad.

13. Stuffed Bell Peppers with Quinoa and Black Beans:

- Ingredients: Bell peppers, quinoa, black beans, corn, salsa.
- Method: Stuff peppers with a mixture of quinoa, black beans, corn, and salsa, then bake.

14. Lentil and Vegetable Curry:

- Ingredients: Lentils, carrots, spinach, coconut milk, curry spices.
- Method: Simmer lentils and vegetables in a coconut milk-based curry sauce.

15. Baked Chicken with Rosemary and Potatoes:

- Ingredients: Chicken thighs, potatoes, rosemary, olive oil.
- Method: Season chicken and potatoes with rosemary and olive oil, bake until golden.

These recipes offer a variety of flavors and textures while prioritizing kidney function. Adjustments can be made based on individual dietary requirements, and it's always advisable to consult with healthcare professionals for personalized guidance.

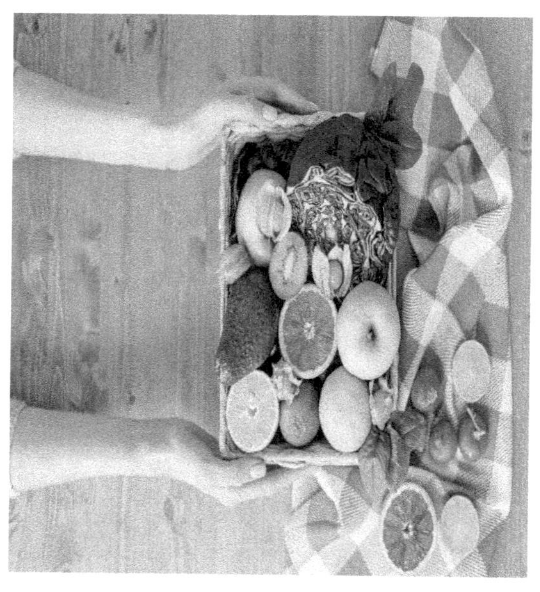

CHAPTER EIGHT

<u>SNACKS AND SIDES FOR SATISFYING CRAVINGS</u>

- **Tempting Bites without Compromising Renal Goals**

Creating tempting bites while adhering to renal diet goals is essential for seniors managing kidney health. This renal diet cookbook focuses on flavorful recipes that prioritize renal-friendly ingredients without compromising on taste.

Recipe 1: Grilled Lemon Herb Chicken
Ingredients:

Chicken breasts
Lemon juice
Fresh herbs (rosemary, thyme)
Olive oil
Instructions:
Marinate chicken in lemon juice, herbs, and olive oil.
Grill until fully cooked.
Accompany with a side order of steaming veggies.

Recipe 2: Quinoa and Vegetable Stir-Fry
Ingredients:

Quinoa
Mixed vegetables (bell peppers, broccoli, carrots)
Low-sodium soy sauce
Garlic
Instructions:
Cook quinoa and stir-fry vegetables with garlic. Add
low-sodium soy sauce for flavor. Combine with
cooked quinoa.

Recipe 3: Baked Salmon with Dill
Ingredients:

Salmon fillets
Fresh dill
Lemon slices
Olive oil
Instructions:
Place salmon on a baking sheet. Drizzle with olive oil,
top with dill and lemon slices. Bake until salmon
flakes easily.

Recipe 4: Creamy Cauliflower Mash
Ingredients:

Cauliflower
Low-fat cream cheese
Garlic powder
Salt and pepper
Instructions:

Steam cauliflower, blend with cream cheese, garlic powder, salt, and pepper. Create a creamy mash as a kidney-friendly alternative to mashed potatoes.

Recipe 5: Turkey and Vegetable Skewers
Ingredients:

Turkey breast chunks
Cherry tomatoes
Zucchini slices
Olive oil
Instructions:
Thread turkey, tomatoes, and zucchini onto skewers. Grill until turkey is cooked. Drizzle with olive oil.

Recipe 6: Spinach and Feta Stuffed Mushrooms
Ingredients:

Mushrooms
Spinach
Feta cheese
Onion
Instructions:
Sauté spinach and onion, mix with crumbled feta. Stuff mushrooms and bake until tender.

Recipe 7: Berry and Yogurt Parfait
Ingredients:

Mixed berries
Low-fat yogurt
Granola
Instructions:

Layer berries, yogurt, and granola for a delicious and kidney-friendly parfait.

Recipe 8: Eggplant and Tomato Casserole
Ingredients:

Eggplant slices
Tomato slices
Low-fat mozzarella
Basil
Instructions:
Layer eggplant and tomato, top with mozzarella and basil. Bake until bubbly.

Recipe 9: Cucumber and Avocado Salad
Ingredients:

Cucumber
Avocado
Red onion
Lemon dressing
Instructions:
Toss sliced cucumber, avocado, and red onion. Drizzle with a light lemon dressing.

Recipe 10: Sweet Potato and Black Bean Chili
Ingredients:

Sweet potatoes
Black beans
Tomatoes
Chili powder
Instructions:

Simmer diced sweet potatoes, black beans, tomatoes, and chili powder for a hearty chili.

Recipe 11: Lemon Garlic Shrimp Skewers
Ingredients:

- Shrimp
- Lemon zest
- Garlic
- Olive oil

Instructions:

Marinate shrimp in lemon zest, minced garlic, and olive oil. Skewer and grill until shrimp turn pink.

Recipe 12: Asparagus and Almond Pilaf

Ingredients:

- Brown rice
- Asparagus spears
- Almonds

- Vegetable broth

Instructions:

Cook brown rice in vegetable broth, stir in blanched asparagus and toasted almonds for a nutty pilaf.

Recipe 13: Chicken and Vegetable Curry

Ingredients:

- Chicken thighs
- Mixed vegetables (bell peppers, peas)
- Curry spices
- Coconut milk

Instructions:

Simmer chicken, vegetables, and curry spices in coconut milk until flavors meld.

Recipe 14: Zesty Orange Glazed Carrots

Ingredients:

- Carrots
- Orange juice
- Honey
- Ginger

Instructions:

Glaze carrots with a mixture of fresh orange juice, honey, and grated ginger. Roast until tender.

Recipe 15: Greek Salad with Chicken

Ingredients:

- Grilled chicken breast
- Cherry tomatoes
- Cucumbers
- Feta cheese

- Olives

Instructions:

Toss grilled chicken, cherry tomatoes, cucumbers, feta, and olives in a light vinaigrette for a refreshing salad.

Recipe 16: Baked Cod with Herbed Tomatoes

Ingredients:

- Cod fillets
- Tomatoes
- Fresh herbs (parsley, basil)
- Lemon juice

Instructions:

Top cod with sliced tomatoes, fresh herbs, and a drizzle of lemon juice. Bake until fish is flaky.

Recipe 17: Roasted Brussels Sprouts with
Cranberries

Ingredients:

- Brussels sprouts
- Dried cranberries
- Balsamic glaze

Instructions:

Roast Brussels sprouts and cranberries, drizzle
with balsamic glaze for a sweet and savory side.

Recipe 18: Lentil and Vegetable Soup

Ingredients:

- Lentils
- Mixed vegetables (carrots, celery, onions)
- Low-sodium vegetable broth
- Herbs (thyme, bay leaves)

Instructions:

Simmer lentils, mixed vegetables, and herbs in low-sodium vegetable broth for a hearty soup.

Recipe 19: Blueberry Oat Muffins

Ingredients:

- Oats
- Blueberries
- Greek yogurt
- Egg whites

Instructions:

Combine oats, blueberries, Greek yogurt, and egg whites to bake delicious and kidney-friendly muffins.

Recipe 20: Vanilla Chia Seed Pudding

Ingredients:

- Chia seeds
- Almond milk
- Vanilla extract
- Fresh berries

Instructions:

Mix chia seeds, almond milk, and vanilla extract.

Refrigerate until it forms a pudding-like consistency.

Top with fresh berries before serving.

Conclusion:

These additional recipes expand the variety of tempting bites for seniors on a renal diet, ensuring a delightful culinary experience without compromising kidney health. Enjoy the rich flavors and textures while adhering to renal goals for overall well-being.

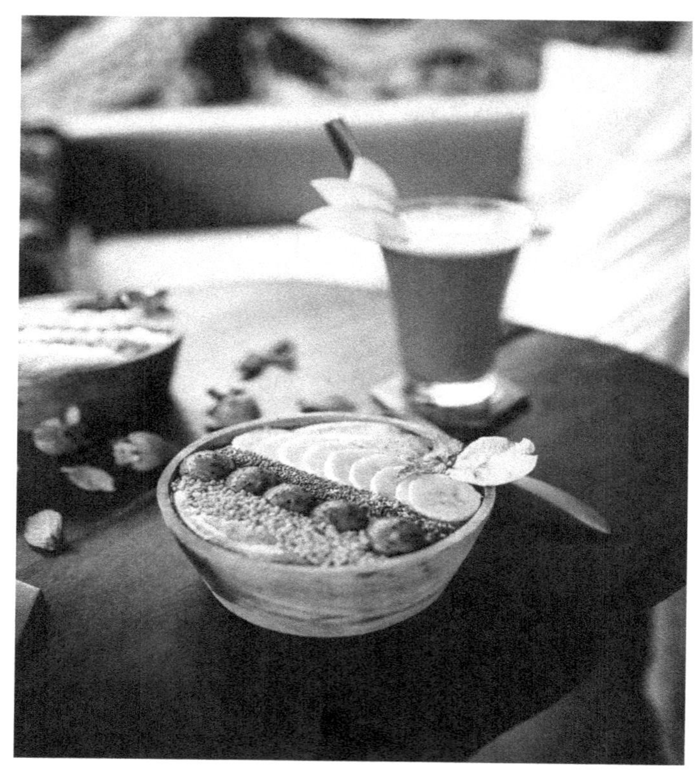

CHAPTER NINE

DESSERTS: SWEET INDULGENCES WITHOUT COMPROMISING HEALTH

- Delectable Treats for a Renal-Friendly Sweet Tooth

1. Chia Seed Pudding with Berries:

Ingredients:

1/4 cup chia seeds

1 cup almond milk (low phosphorus)

1 tsp vanilla extract

Mixed berries (blueberries, strawberries)

Instructions:

In a dish, combine almond milk, vanilla essence, and chia seeds.

Let it sit in the fridge for at least 2 hours or overnight.

Top with fresh mixed berries before serving.

2. Baked Apple Slices:

Ingredients:

2 apples, cored and sliced

1 tsp cinnamon

1 tbsp honey

Instructions:

Preheat oven to 375°F (190°C).

Toss apple slices with cinnamon and honey.

Bake apples for 20 to 25 minutes, or until they are soft.

3. Frozen Yogurt Bites:

Ingredients:

1 cup low-phosphorus yogurt

1 tbsp honey

Fresh fruit (e.g., diced peaches)

Instructions:

Mix yogurt and honey.

Spoon small dollops onto a tray.

Top with diced fruit and freeze for a few hours.

4. Almond Flour Banana Muffins:

Ingredients:

2 ripe bananas, mashed

1 cup almond flour

1/4 cup honey

1 tsp baking powder

Instructions:

Preheat oven to 350°F (175°C).

Mix mashed bananas, almond flour, honey, and

baking powder.

Pour into muffin cups and bake for 20-25 minutes.

5. Vanilla Rice Pudding:

Ingredients:

1/2 cup white rice

2 cups low-phosphorus milk

1/4 cup sugar

1 tsp vanilla extract

Instructions:

Cook rice in milk until tender.

Stir in sugar and vanilla extract.

Chill before serving.

6. Cranberry Orange Sorbet:

Ingredients:

2 cups fresh cranberries

1 cup water

1/2 cup orange juice

1/4 cup sugar

Instructions:

Boil cranberries, water, and sugar until berries burst.

Blend with orange juice and freeze in a pan.

Fluff with a fork before serving.

Conclusion:

These renal-friendly desserts are not only delicious but also considerate of dietary restrictions. Always get the counsel of a medical expert before making any dietary changes.

Enjoy these treats guilt-free while maintaining kidney health!

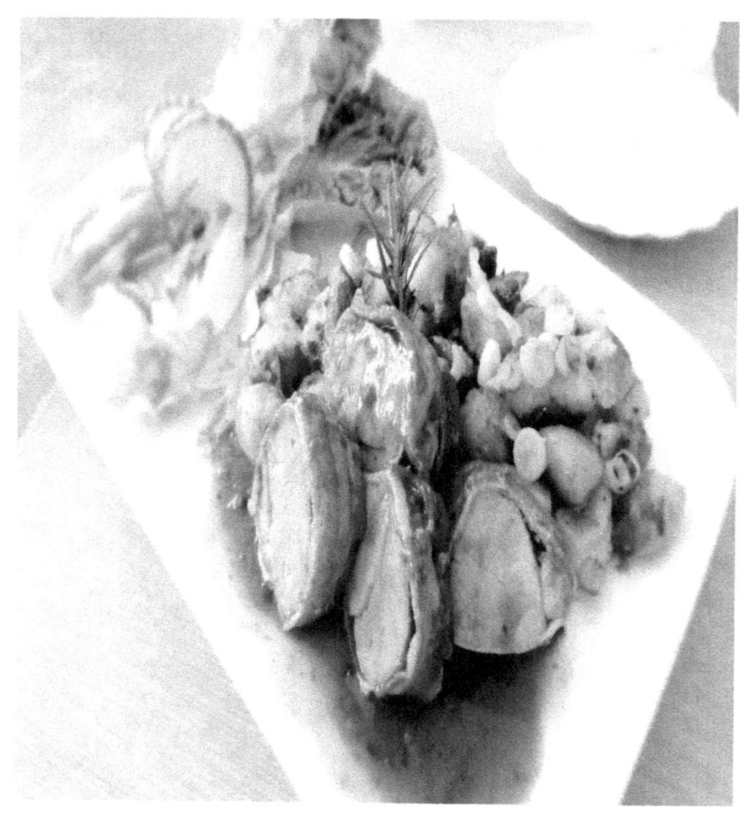

CHAPTER TEN

BEVERAGES FOR HYDRATION AND KIDNEY SUPPORT

- Refreshing Drinks to Boost Kidney Function

Lemonade with Fresh Mint:

Lemonade is a hydrating and low-calorie option that can be kidney-friendly. Citrate, which is found in lemons, may help avoid kidney stones.

Add fresh mint for a burst of flavor and potential antioxidant benefits.

Cucumber and Watermelon Infused Water:

Both cucumber and watermelon have high water content, promoting hydration and supporting kidney function.

Cucumber is known for its diuretic properties, assisting in flushing out toxins.

Herbal Tea Blend:
Certain herbal teas, such as dandelion or nettle tea, are believed to have mild diuretic effects and can aid in kidney function.
Choose caffeine-free options to avoid dehydration.

Cranberry Juice (Unsweetened):
Unsweetened cranberry juice may help prevent urinary tract infections, promoting overall kidney health.
Ensure it is low in added sugars, as excessive sugar intake can negatively impact kidney function.

Ginger Turmeric Tea:
Ginger and turmeric both have anti-inflammatory properties and are thought to have potential benefits for kidney health.
Brew a warm tea using fresh ginger and turmeric for a soothing beverage.

Coconut Water:

Coconut water is a natural electrolyte-rich drink that can aid in hydration.

It is low in potassium, making it a suitable choice for those with kidney concerns.

Blueberry Smoothie:

Blueberries are rich in antioxidants and may have anti-inflammatory effects that could support kidney health.

Blend fresh or frozen blueberries with a low-potassium base like almond milk.

Pomegranate Juice:

Pomegranates are rich in antioxidants and may have potential kidney-protective effects.

Opt for pure pomegranate juice without added sugars for the best benefits.

Chamomile Lemonade:

Chamomile tea is known for its calming properties and may have mild diuretic effects.

Combine it with fresh lemon juice for a kidney-friendly twist on classic lemonade.

Minty Green Tea:

Green tea is a hydrating option with potential antioxidant properties.

Add fresh mint leaves to enhance the flavor and add a refreshing twist.

Recipes And Instructions

Lemonade with Fresh Mint:
Ingredients: Freshly squeezed lemon juice, water, mint leaves, honey (optional).
Instructions: Mix 1 cup of lemon juice with 4 cups of water. Add crushed mint leaves and sweeten with honey if desired. Stir well and serve over ice.

Cucumber and Watermelon Infused Water:
Ingredients: Sliced cucumber, cubed watermelon, water.
Instructions: Combine cucumber slices and watermelon cubes in a pitcher of water. Refrigerate for a few hours. Serve over ice.

Herbal Tea Blend:

Ingredients: Dandelion or nettle tea bags, hot water.
Instructions: Steep dandelion or nettle tea bags in hot water for 5-7 minutes. Remove the bags and enjoy the herbal tea.

Cranberry Juice (Unsweetened):
Ingredients: Unsweetened cranberry juice, water.
Instructions: Dilute unsweetened cranberry juice with water to taste. Serve chilled over ice.

Ginger Turmeric Tea:
Ingredients: Fresh ginger, fresh turmeric, hot water.
Instructions: Grate ginger and turmeric into hot water... After ten minutes of steeping, strain and serve.

Coconut Water:
Ingredients: Fresh coconut water.
Instructions: Chill fresh coconut water and serve it over ice for a hydrating experience.

Blueberry Smoothie:
Ingredients: Fresh or frozen blueberries, low-potassium base (almond milk), natural sweetener.
Instructions: Blend blueberries with almond milk and sweeten to taste. Pour over ice.

Pomegranate Juice:
Ingredients: Fresh pomegranate seeds or store-bought pure pomegranate juice.
Instructions: Extract juice from fresh seeds or use pure pomegranate juice. Serve chilled.

Chamomile Lemonade:
Ingredients: Chamomile tea bags, freshly squeezed lemon juice, water, natural sweetener.
Instructions: Steep chamomile tea bags in hot water. Mix with lemon juice, sweeten to taste, and serve over ice.

Minty Green Tea:
Ingredients: Green tea bags, fresh mint leaves, hot water.
Instructions: Steep green tea bags and mint leaves in hot water for 3-5 minutes. Remove the bags and mint before serving.
Feel free to customize these recipes based on personal preferences, adjusting sweetness or dilution to suit individual taste.

CHAPTER ELEVEN

MEAL PLANNING TIPS AND TRICKS

- Practical Strategies for a Renal-Optimized Diet.

A renal-optimized diet is crucial for individuals with kidney-related concerns, aiming to manage their condition through thoughtful food choices. Meal planning plays a pivotal role in maintaining a balanced and kidney-friendly diet. Here are practical strategies to help you navigate the complexities of meal planning for renal health.

**1. ** Monitor Phosphorus and Potassium Intake:

Focus on foods with lower phosphorus and potassium levels. This includes choosing white bread over whole wheat, and cooking vegetables in water to reduce potassium content.

**2. ** Limit Sodium Intake:
Limit your intake of packaged and processed foods because they frequently have high salt content.
 Opt for fresh ingredients and use herbs and spices for flavor instead of salt.

**3. ** Manage Protein Intake:

Consult with a healthcare professional to determine an appropriate protein level for your condition. Include high-quality protein sources like lean meats, fish, and eggs in moderation.

**4. ** Plan Portion Sizes:

Control portion sizes to avoid overloading the kidneys. Use smaller plates to help manage portions effectively, preventing excessive intake of nutrients that may strain kidney function.

**5. ** Prioritize Plant-Based Proteins:

Add sources of plant-based protein including tofu, lentils, and beans.

These alternatives provide essential nutrients without placing excessive stress on the kidneys.

**6. ** Stay Hydrated:

Adequate hydration is vital for kidney health. Monitor fluid intake based on your individual needs and consult with your healthcare provider to determine the right amount for you.

**7. ** Choose Low-Phosphorus Grains:

Opt for grains with lower phosphorus content, such as rice, pasta, and corn. This helps in managing phosphorus levels while still enjoying staple foods.

**8. ** Plan Balanced Meals:

Create well-rounded meals that include a mix of carbohydrates, proteins, and fats. This ensures a diverse nutrient intake without overloading specific components that may be problematic for kidney function.

**9. ** Experiment with Cooking Techniques:

Explore various cooking methods to enhance flavors without compromising nutritional integrity. Grilling, roasting, and steaming are great alternatives to frying, which may introduce additional unhealthy elements.

**10. ** Read Food Labels:
- Scrutinize food labels for phosphorus, potassium, and sodium content. Being informed about the nutritional composition of packaged foods aids in making kidney-friendly choices.

**11. ** Snack Smartly:

- Opt for renal-friendly snacks, such as fresh fruits, raw vegetables, and low-phosphorus crackers. This helps maintain consistent nutrient intake throughout the day.

**12. ** Consult a Renal Dietitian:
- Work closely with a renal dietitian to create a personalized meal plan. A professional can offer tailored advice based on your specific dietary needs, helping you manage your renal health effectively.

**13. ** Plan Ahead for Dining Out:
- Research restaurant menus in advance to make informed choices. Communicate your dietary restrictions to the staff, and consider ordering sauces and dressings on the side to control intake.

**14. ** Be Mindful of Hidden Phosphorus:
- Some foods may contain hidden phosphorus additives. Avoiding processed and convenience foods helps reduce the risk of unintentional phosphorus overload.

**15. ** Include Essential Nutrients:

- Ensure your diet includes essential nutrients like calcium and vitamin D. While these should be moderated, they are important for overall health and can be supplemented if necessary.

Day 1:

Breakfast: Oatmeal made with water, topped with sliced strawberries and a sprinkle of chopped almonds.
Lunch: Grilled chicken breast with steamed green beans and quinoa.
Dinner: Baked salmon, brown rice, and sautéed spinach.
Day 2:

Breakfast: Scrambled eggs with diced bell peppers and whole-grain toast.
Lunch: Lentil soup with a side of mixed greens and a lemon vinaigrette.
Dinner: Stir-fried tofu with broccoli and cauliflower over white rice.
Day 3:

Greek yogurt topped with honey and a few blueberries for breakfast.
Lunch: Turkey and vegetable wrap with a whole-grain tortilla.

Dinner: Grilled shrimp with quinoa and roasted asparagus.
Day 4:

Breakfast: Smoothie made with banana, low-phosphorus protein powder, and almond milk.
Lunch: Chickpea salad with cherry tomatoes, cucumber, and a light olive oil dressing.
Dinner: Baked chicken thighs with sweet potato wedges and steamed peas.
Day 5:
Breakfast is sliced peaches and cottage cheese with a dash of sunflower seeds.

Lunch: Spinach and feta stuffed chicken breast with a side of couscous.
Dinner: Cod fish tacos with cabbage slaw and a side of black beans.
Day 6:

Breakfast: Whole-grain waffle topped with low-potassium fruit compote.
Lunch: Quinoa salad with cherry tomatoes, cucumbers, and grilled zucchini.
Dinner: Stir-fried beef strips with bell peppers and brown rice.
Day 7:

Breakfast: Poached eggs over avocado toast with a side of melon.
Lunch: Shredded chicken salad with mixed greens, cherry tomatoes, and a balsamic vinaigrette.

Dinner: Baked trout with wild rice and steamed broccoli.

Remember to drink water throughout the day to stay adequately hydrated. Adjust portion sizes and specific food choices based on individual dietary restrictions and preferences. This sample meal plan is a general guide and may need modification based on your unique health considerations.

 Seek individual counsel from healthcare specialists at all times.

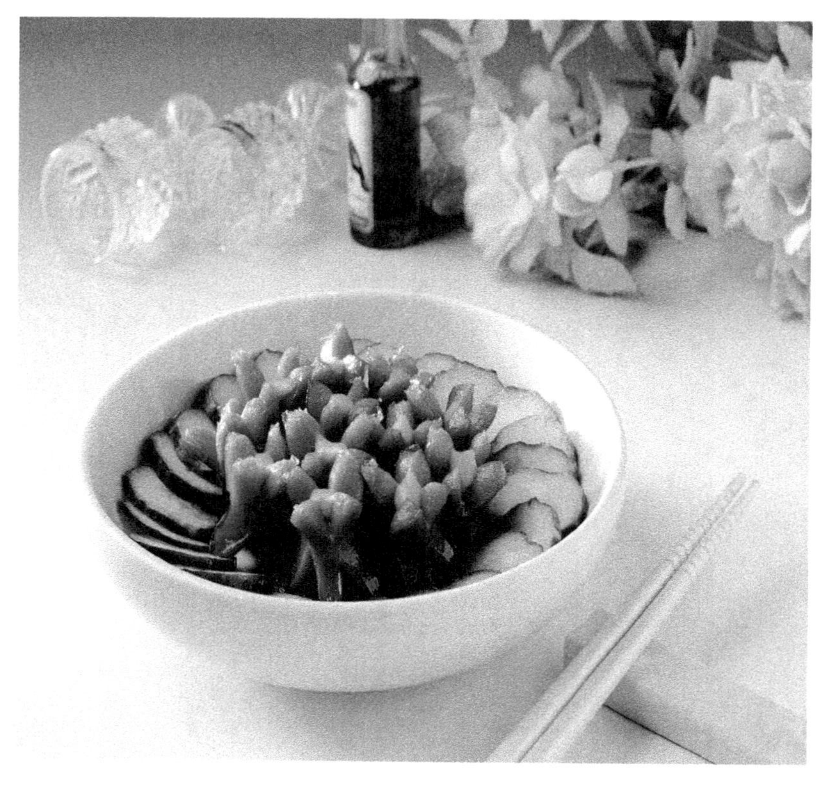

CHAPTER TWELVE

MANAGING DINING OUT: A GUIDE FOR SENIORS

- **Navigating Restaurants with Renal Health in Mind**

Maintaining renal health requires careful consideration of dietary choices, and this becomes particularly crucial when dining out at restaurants. For individuals with kidney issues, managing sodium, potassium, and phosphorus intake is essential to prevent further complications. Navigating restaurant menus with renal health in mind involves making informed choices, communicating with restaurant staff, and being mindful of specific dietary restrictions.

Understanding Renal Dietary Restrictions

Before delving into strategies for navigating restaurant menus, it's crucial to understand the dietary restrictions associated with renal health. Individuals with kidney problems often need to limit their intake of sodium, potassium, and phosphorus. Excessive sodium can contribute to high blood pressure, while elevated levels of potassium and phosphorus may strain the kidneys. Therefore, a renal-friendly diet focuses on controlling these elements without compromising overall nutrition.

Strategies for Navigating Restaurant Menus

Researching Restaurants in Advance: Before heading to a restaurant, research its menu online. Many establishments now provide nutritional information, allowing you to assess sodium, potassium, and phosphorus content. Opt for restaurants that offer customizable options or have a variety of dishes suitable for renal diets.

Choosing Lean Proteins: When selecting protein sources, opt for lean options such as grilled chicken, fish, or lean cuts of meat. These choices are not only lower in saturated fat but also help manage phosphorus intake, which can be high in certain protein-rich foods.

Requesting Modifications: Don't hesitate to request modifications to your dish. Ask for sauces, dressings, or toppings on the side, allowing you to control the amount you consume. Most restaurants are accommodating to dietary requests, and chefs are often willing to adjust recipes to meet specific needs.

Being Wary of Hidden Sodium: Restaurant meals can be laden with hidden sodium. Avoid dishes that are heavily processed, fried, or overly seasoned. Instead, opt for fresh, grilled, or steamed options. Additionally, inquire about low-sodium alternatives or ask if the chef can prepare your meal with minimal salt.

Monitoring Portion Sizes: Renal health is closely tied to maintaining a healthy weight. Many restaurants serve larger portions than necessary, contributing to overconsumption of nutrients. Consider sharing a meal or requesting a smaller portion size to manage your intake effectively.

Choosing Side Dishes Wisely: Side dishes can significantly impact the overall nutritional content of a meal. Opt for renal-friendly sides like steamed vegetables or a baked potato without excessive toppings. Be cautious of sides that may be high in sodium, such as seasoned rice or fries.

Limiting High-Potassium Foods: Bananas, oranges, tomatoes, and potatoes are high-potassium foods that should be consumed in moderation. When dining out, be mindful of dishes that may contain these ingredients and consider alternatives to keep potassium levels in check.

Hydrating Smartly: Proper hydration is essential for kidney health. Choose water, herbal tea, or other low-potassium beverages over sodas or high-potassium fruit juices. Be cautious of alcohol, which can dehydrate the body, and limit its consumption.

Communicating with Restaurant Staff

Effective communication with restaurant staff is key to ensuring your dietary needs are met. Don't hesitate to inform your server about your renal restrictions and ask questions about the preparation methods used. Most restaurants are willing to accommodate dietary requests and can provide valuable insights into menu options suitable for renal health.

Additionally, expressing gratitude for their assistance can foster a positive relationship, encouraging staff to be more attentive to your specific needs. Remember that your health is a priority, and a proactive approach to communication can make dining out a more enjoyable and stress-free experience.

Conclusion

Navigating restaurants with renal health in mind requires a combination of research, careful menu selection, and effective communication with restaurant staff. By understanding and adhering to renal dietary restrictions, individuals can make informed choices to support their kidney health while still enjoying dining out. Embracing a proactive approach and staying mindful of portion sizes and hidden sodium are integral steps toward maintaining a renal-friendly diet. With these strategies, individuals can confidently navigate restaurant menus, making choices that align with their health goals and contribute to overall well-being.

CHAPTER THIRTEEN

<u>LIFESTYLE HABITS FOR</u>

<u>IMPROVED RENAL FUNCTION</u>

- Beyond the Plate: Holistic Approaches to Kidney Health.

Kidney health extends beyond dietary considerations alone; adopting a holistic approach that encompasses lifestyle, mental well-being, and overall health is crucial for promoting optimal renal function. While a renal-friendly diet is foundational, incorporating holistic practices can provide a comprehensive approach to supporting kidney health and preventing complications. Here are key aspects to consider beyond the plate:

1. Hydration and Kidney Function:

Proper hydration is fundamental for kidney health.Water supports healthy kidney function by removing waste materials and poisons from the body, which helps avoid kidney stones from forming. Adequate hydration also helps maintain optimal blood flow to the kidneys.

Incorporate the habit of drinking water throughout the day. While individual water needs vary, a general guideline is to aim for at least 8 cups (64 ounces) daily. You may increase your regular fluid intake by consuming herbal teas and fruits and vegetables that are high in water.

2. Regular Physical Activity:

Exercise plays a pivotal role in maintaining overall health, and it can positively impact kidney function. Regular physical activity helps control blood pressure, manage weight, and improve cardiovascular health – factors directly linked to kidney well-being.

Take up exercises like cycling, swimming, or walking. As advised by health recommendations, aim for at least 150 minutes a week of moderate-intensity exercise. Before beginning a new fitness program, always get medical advice, especially if you have any underlying medical issues.

3. Blood Pressure Management:

Kidney injury is mostly caused by high blood pressure.Adopting lifestyle changes to manage blood pressure is crucial for kidney health.Limit salt consumption, keep a healthy weight, and work out frequently.Additionally, limit alcohol consumption and quit smoking, as these habits can elevate blood pressure.

Monitoring blood pressure regularly and working closely with healthcare professionals to manage hypertension is essential. Medication adherence, if prescribed, is a vital component of a comprehensive strategy to protect kidney function.

4. Stress Reduction Techniques:

Chronic stress can contribute to a variety of health issues, including kidney problems. Implementing stress reduction techniques can positively impact overall well-being. Practices such as mindfulness meditation, deep breathing exercises, and yoga can help manage stress levels.

Finding activities that bring joy and relaxation is also important. Whether it's reading, listening to music, or spending time in nature, incorporating these activities into your routine can contribute to a holistic approach to kidney health.

5. Adequate Sleep:

Quality sleep is essential for overall health, and it plays a role in supporting kidney function. During sleep, the body undergoes important processes, including the removal of waste products. Chronic sleep deprivation can lead to impaired kidney function and increase the risk of developing kidney disease.

Establish a regular sleep schedule, create a comfortable sleep environment, and prioritize sufficient sleep each night. If sleep issues persist, consult with a healthcare professional for guidance.

6. Avoiding Over-the-Counter Medications:

Certain over-the-counter medications, when used excessively, can contribute to kidney damage. Nonsteroidal anti-inflammatory drugs (NSAIDs) like ibuprofen and naproxen can be particularly harmful. Consult with a healthcare provider before regularly using such medications, especially if you have pre-existing kidney conditions.

7. Regular Health Check-ups:

Regular health check-ups are crucial for identifying potential kidney issues early on. Routine blood pressure monitoring, urine tests, and blood tests can provide valuable insights into kidney function. Detecting and addressing problems in their early stages can significantly improve outcomes and prevent further complications.

Conclusion:

Adopting a holistic approach to kidney health goes beyond dietary choices. By integrating practices such as proper hydration, regular exercise, stress reduction, adequate sleep, and avoiding harmful medications, individuals can promote overall well-being and support optimal kidney function. Regular health check-ups provide an opportunity for early detection and intervention, further enhancing the effectiveness of a holistic approach to kidney health. Remember that lifestyle changes should be implemented in consultation with healthcare professionals to ensure they align with individual health needs and conditions. Embracing these holistic practices empowers individuals to take proactive steps towards maintaining kidney health and enjoying a vibrant and fulfilling life.

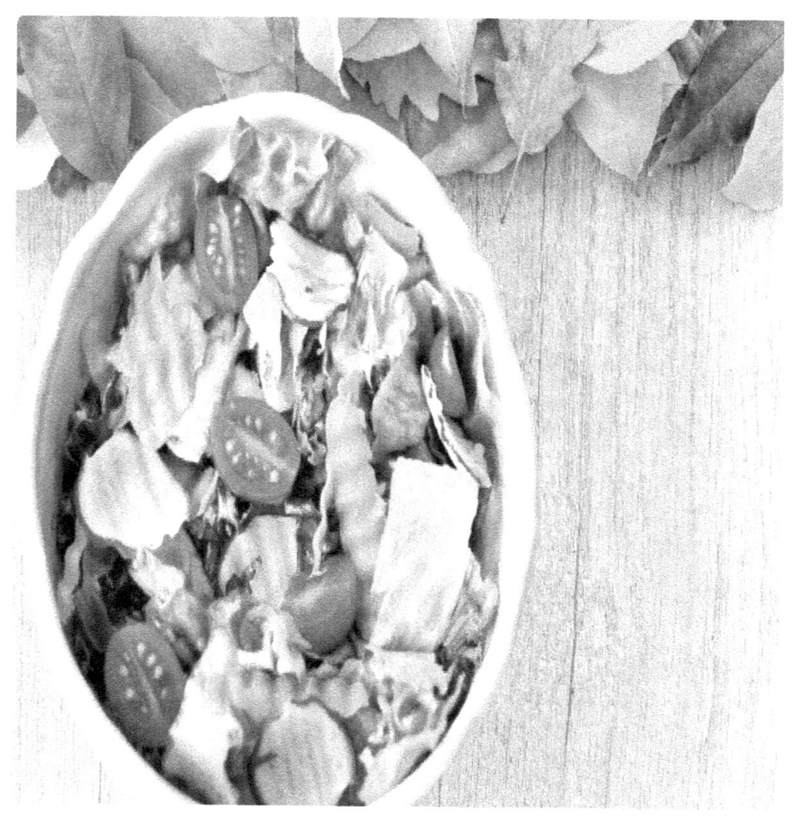

CHAPTER FOURTEEN

RECIPES AT A GLANCE: QUICK REFERENCE GUIDE

- Easy Access to Your Favorite Renal-Friendly Dishes

Ensuring a renal-friendly diet is accessible and enjoyable is essential for individuals managing kidney health. With a bit of planning, awareness, and creativity, one can easily access and relish a variety of renal-friendly dishes. From home-cooked meals to dining out, here's a comprehensive guide to making renal-friendly eating a seamless part of daily life.

**1. Home-Cooked Delights:

Meal Planning:

Begin by planning your meals to include a balance of nutrients while adhering to renal dietary restrictions. Focus on incorporating lean proteins, limited sodium, and controlled portions of high-potassium and high-phosphorus foods. Consider consulting a registered dietitian to create personalized meal plans that align with your specific renal needs.

Fresh Ingredients:
Opt for fresh fruits and vegetables, lean meats, and whole grains. Fresh produce is not only rich in essential nutrients but also allows you to control the amount of sodium and other additives in your meals. Experiment with a variety of herbs and spices to enhance flavor without relying on salt.

Smart Cooking Methods:
Choose cooking methods that retain the nutritional value of your ingredients. Grilling, baking, steaming, and sautéing are healthier alternatives to frying. These methods help preserve the natural flavors of foods without adding unnecessary fats or sodium.

**2. Renal-Friendly Recipes:

Explore Recipe Books and Websites:
There are numerous cookbooks and websites dedicated to renal-friendly recipes. These resources provide a wealth of ideas for delicious dishes that align with dietary restrictions. From flavorful salads to satisfying main courses, you can discover a variety of recipes catering to different tastes and preferences.

Ingredient Substitutions:
Get creative with ingredient substitutions to make your favorite recipes renal-friendly. For example, swap high-potassium potatoes with lower-potassium alternatives like sweet potatoes. Experimenting with alternatives allows you to adapt recipes while maintaining nutritional balance.

Meal Prepping:

Consider incorporating meal prepping into your routine. Preparing meals in advance not only saves time but also ensures that you have renal-friendly options readily available. Portion out meals into containers, making it convenient to grab a nutritious option when needed.

**3. Dining Out with Confidence:

Menu Exploration:
Before heading to a restaurant, explore the menu online or call ahead to inquire about renal-friendly options. Many establishments are willing to accommodate dietary needs, and some may even have a separate section on their menu for healthier choices.

Communication with Staff:

Don't hesitate to communicate with restaurant staff about your dietary restrictions. Inform your server about your renal needs, and ask for modifications to suit your requirements. Most chefs are willing to adjust recipes or customize dishes to make them renal-friendly.

Focus on Lean Proteins:
When dining out, opt for dishes centered around lean proteins such as grilled chicken, fish, or lean cuts of meat. These choices not only align with renal dietary guidelines but also contribute to a well-balanced and satisfying meal.

Sides Matter:
Be mindful of side dishes, as they can significantly impact the overall nutritional content of your meal. Choose sides like steamed vegetables or a small salad to complement your main dish while keeping sodium and potassium levels in check.

**4. Online Resources and Apps:

Nutritional Apps:

Utilize nutritional apps that provide information about the nutritional content of various foods. These apps can help you track your daily intake of sodium, potassium, and phosphorus, ensuring you stay within recommended limits. Some apps also offer renal-specific tracking features.

Recipe Apps and Websites:

Explore recipe apps and websites that focus on renal-friendly dishes. These platforms often offer filters or categories specifically designed for individuals managing kidney health. You can discover new recipes, save favorites, and even create shopping lists to streamline your cooking experience.

**5. Community Support and Tips:

Online Communities:

Joining online communities or forums dedicated to renal health can provide valuable insights and support. Share your experiences, learn from others, and exchange tips on accessing and enjoying renal-friendly dishes. These communities often offer a sense of camaraderie and encouragement on the journey to better kidney health.

Local Support Groups:
Look for local support groups or workshops that focus on renal health and nutrition. Connecting with individuals facing similar challenges can be both informative and uplifting. Attendees often share tips on sourcing renal-friendly ingredients and discuss favorite local spots that offer suitable menu options.

Conclusion:

Achieving easy access to your favorite renal-friendly dishes involves a combination of home cooking, exploration of recipes, dining out with confidence, leveraging online resources, and seeking community support. By taking a proactive approach to meal planning, experimenting with ingredients, and utilizing technology and community connections, individuals managing kidney health can enjoy a diverse and satisfying array of meals. Remember, embracing a renal-friendly lifestyle is not about restriction but about making informed choices that contribute to overall well-being and a delicious, nourishing dining experience.

CONCLUSION

The significance of a renal diet cookbook for seniors cannot be overstated. As we navigate the intricacies of aging, it becomes imperative to prioritize our health, particularly when faced with renal challenges. The culmination of knowledge, culinary expertise, and nutritional wisdom encapsulated within a renal diet cookbook offers seniors not just a collection of recipes, but a roadmap to better well-being.

The essence of a renal diet lies in its ability to empower seniors with the tools to manage their kidney health proactively. The cookbook serves as a comprehensive guide, acknowledging the unique dietary needs of aging individuals grappling with renal issues. It amalgamates flavors, textures, and nutritional elements in a way that transcends the conventional notion of restricted diets, transforming them into a gastronomic adventure tailored to nourish both body and soul.

One cannot underscore the importance of variety in a renal diet cookbook enough. The diverse array of recipes ensures that seniors are not only meeting their nutritional requirements but also relishing their meals. From tantalizing appetizers to hearty main courses and delectable desserts, the cookbook cultivates a sense of culinary exploration. It dispels the notion that a renal diet is monotonous, proving that health-conscious meals can be both palatable and satisfying.

Furthermore, the renal diet cookbook fosters an understanding of the intricate relationship between food and renal health. Seniors are not merely following recipes; they are engaging in a transformative learning experience. The cookbook becomes a trusted companion, imparting knowledge about the nutritional value of ingredients, the impact of cooking methods, and the significance of portion control. This knowledge empowers seniors to make informed choices, fostering a sense of autonomy and control over their health.

Beyond the kitchen, the renal diet cookbook extends its influence to the broader aspects of seniors' lives. It promotes a holistic approach to well-being by encouraging an active lifestyle, hydration, and mindful eating. The cookbook is a catalyst for a paradigm shift – from viewing a renal diet as a restrictive measure to perceiving it as a gateway to vitality. It becomes a tool not just for managing renal health but for enhancing overall quality of life.

Importantly, the cookbook transcends generational barriers. It serves as a testament to the adaptability of culinary traditions, demonstrating that age should not be a deterrent to savoring delicious, health-conscious meals. It bridges the gap between generations, fostering a shared appreciation for the importance of good nutrition. In doing so, it lays the foundation for a healthier future, where the wisdom of balanced eating is passed down from one generation to the next.

In a world inundated with fad diets and quick fixes, the renal diet cookbook stands as a beacon of evidence-based nutrition. It dispels misconceptions and guides seniors towards sustainable, long-term health. It is a celebration of the body's resilience and the transformative power of wholesome, nourishing food.

In conclusion, a renal diet cookbook for seniors is not merely a compilation of recipes; it is a comprehensive guide to embracing and optimizing health in the later years of life. It symbolizes a commitment to well-being, a journey of culinary discovery, and a testament to the power of informed choices. As seniors embark on this gastronomic adventure, armed with the knowledge and flavors encapsulated within the cookbook, they are not just cooking; they are crafting a legacy of health, vitality, and longevity.

THANK YOU

As we reach the culmination of this culinary journey, I want to express my deepest gratitude for joining me on the pages of the "Renal Diet Cookbook for Seniors." Your dedication to exploring the transformative power of health-conscious and flavorful meals is truly appreciated.

Thank you for entrusting me with a small part of your kitchen adventures. It's my sincere hope that this cookbook has not only filled your table with delicious and nourishing dishes but also enriched your understanding of the profound connection between food and well-being. Your commitment to embracing a renal-friendly lifestyle is a commendable step towards a healthier, more vibrant you.

In every recipe shared, every nutritional tip offered, and every culinary adventure embarked upon, your enthusiasm for prioritizing your health shines through. The pages of this cookbook serve as a testament to your dedication to a wholesome and fulfilling life. As you savor each carefully crafted dish, may it bring joy, vitality, and a sense of empowerment to your daily routine.

Remember, this journey is not just about recipes; it's a celebration of the choices we make for our health and the joy we derive from mindful, delicious meals. So, from the bottom of my heart, thank you for making "Renal Diet Cookbook for Seniors" a part of your culinary repertoire. May your kitchen continue to be a place of nourishment, experimentation, and joy.

Wishing you vibrant health and countless delightful moments in your culinary explorations. Thank you for reading, and here's to the continued joy of cooking and savoring every bite of life's flavorful chapters.